THE 5:2 DIET
FOR BEGINNERS

A Quick Start Guide to Intermittent Fasting, Rapid Weight Loss, and a Long Healthy Life

Gina Crawford

Evita Publishing, PO Box 306, Station A, Vancouver Island, BC V9W 5B1 Canada

IMPORTANT

The information in this book reflects the author's research, experiences, and opinions and is not intended to replace medical advice.

Before beginning this or any nutritional or exercise regimen, consult your physician to be sure it is appropriate for you. Ask for a physical stress test.

Table of Contents

Introduction

The 5:2 diet can revolutionize the way you think about weight loss and dieting!

Contrary to popular belief, eating six small meals a day can actually hurt you rather than help you according to the founder of the 5:2 diet, Dr. Michael Mosley.

The 5:2 diet focuses on intermittent fasting as a vehicle for weight loss and longevity. Though the diet itself is fairly new, the underlying concept of fasting is backed by over 20 years of research. Scientific research that has been done on intermittent fasting has revealed extraordinary results in the area of life extension, better health, and weight loss. Today, scientists continue to research the benefits of intermittent fasting for weight loss, disease prevention, and longevity.

This book will teach you the ins and outs of the 5:2 diet. It also includes quick and easy 30 minute low glycemic recipes that will make your fast days easier!

If you receive value from this book please consider posting a review on Amazon. Even a one or two line review is helpful and much appreciated. Thanks!

Chapter 1

What is the 5:2 Diet?

"Fasting is the first thing I've come across that I genuinely believe, if people were to take it up, could radically transform the nation's health."

Dr. Michael Mosley

The 5:2 diet, or *fast diet,* is a unique approach to dieting that uses intermittent fasting to promote weight loss and better health. It was popularized in 2012 by Dr. Michael Mosley, a British television journalist, producer, and science presenter.

Though the 5:2 diet itself is fairly new, the concept of fasting and the study of the benefits of fasting on human health are not. Some of the world's leading scientists have been studying the tremendous health benefits of fasting for over 20 years.

The 5:2 diet is unique in that it challenges our understanding of what the right way to diet really is. We've been taught to believe that in order to maintain a healthy lifestyle and lose weight it's important to eat regularly (six small meals a day), avoid getting hungry, consume low-fat foods, and exercise for a minimum of 30 minutes a day.

The 5:2 diet on the other hand, tells you to:

Fast on two non-consecutive days of the week by cutting your calorie intake to about one quarter of what it normally is (500 calories for women, 600 calories for men).

Eat what you want for 5 days a week.

Do a high intensity workout for ten minutes three times a week along with some strength training.

Why does the 5:2 diet work?

The human body was designed to fast

Human beings evolved at a time when feast or famine was the norm. Thousands of years ago, eating three to four meals a day was unheard of. People back then would kill something, eat it, and then eat nothing until they went out again to hunt their next meal. This interim period of not eating caused the body to become stressed at a cellular level, but it was a good kind of stress that prompted the body to go into a repair and maintenance mode which ultimately made the body healthier and tougher. In science this is called hormesis. This process is similar to what happens when you exercise. Muscles get torn and stressed but when you recover, you recover a lot stronger than before you exercised. Fasting on two non-consecutive days intentionally provokes good stress in the body and that promotes better health and weight loss.

You consume less calories

The 5:2 diet works because you consume only one quarter of your regular daily calories two days a week. According to physics, that means you should expect to lose about one pound of fat per week. When you first start the 5:2 diet you will typically look like you've lost more than one pound per week because you'll be losing water. As you continue with the diet you can expect to keep losing about one pound of fat per week without muscle loss.

It's not your typical diet

The 5:2 diet works because it doesn't involve the usual diet dread that comes with knowing you've got eight weeks ahead of you of eating nothing but leaves and carrot sticks. Because the 5:2 diet allows you to eat a chocolate bar if you want it, it lessons your temptation for it.

Plus, eating vegetables and good sources of protein on fast days helps you crave healthy foods more often.

High intensity workouts maximize your efforts

The effectiveness of high intensity workouts is a new evolving field of study. Scientists are changing the current view of exercise by proving that only 3 minutes of high intensity exercise per week can make a dramatic difference. Pairing a high intensity workout with the 5:2 diet boosts your dieting efforts.

There's nothing complicated about it

The 5:2 diet is a straight-forward, easy to implement diet that does not involve awkward and lengthy rules, monotonous calorie counting, or deprivation.

It's a lifestyle

The 5:2 diet will help you lose weight but its long term health benefits will likely entice you to stick with it.

The 5:2 diet decreases your risk of a number of diseases including heart disease, cancer, and diabetes. It promotes a healthy, long, and energetic life.

Chapter 2

Why was the 5:2 Diet Created?

The 5:2 diet was created by Dr. Michael Mosley, a British (non-practicing) general physician. Mosley originally studied medicine with the intention of becoming a psychiatrist but upon graduation changed his focus to television. He went on to produce several science programs for the BBC that covered a wide range of topics from neuroscience to weight loss.

Mosley is well known for his programs that focus on medicine and biology, particularly his series on the workings of the human body, inside the human body.

In 1995 the British Medical Association named Dr. Michael Mosley, Medical Journalist of the Year.

In 2012, Dr. Mosley appeared in the BBC 2 Horizon documentary *Eat, Fast, Live Longer* which had a huge global response. Later that year he was credited with popularizing the 5:2 diet.

Why Dr. Mosley developed the 5:2 diet

Two years prior to popularizing the 5:2 diet, Mosley went to see his doctor for a routine checkup and was unexpectedly diagnosed with diabetes due to his extremely high blood sugar levels. He was also told that his cholesterol level was too high and that he had metabolic syndrome.

Though he didn't appear overweight on the outside he was fat on the inside with visceral fat. Visceral fat is stored in the abdominal cavity (stomach) around important internal organs like the pancreas, liver, and intestines. It can severely increase the risk of developing heart disease and diabetes.

Mosley's doctor wanted to start him on drugs in order to treat his illnesses, but Mosley declined because he was interested in seeing if there was a way to cure his condition without drugs. Shortly after Mosley started researching alternative healing methods he came across the concept of intermittent fasting.

With a keen interest in self-experimentation and testing dieting methods that seemed rather off the wall, he and the editor of the science branch of the BBC (Horizon) agreed to make a film in which he would test intermittent fasting on himself to see if it could improve his health.

At first he tried the regular dieting advice that he was taught as a doctor but it had no significant impact on his health. He then started a calorie restriction diet that involved eating a very small amount of calories every day. He personally found this plan quite difficult and almost impossible to maintain.

He then dove into intermittent fasting and began exploring the different ways in which intermittent fasting could be done. Some methods involved fasting for 24 hours or more. Others involved eating one low calorie meal once every two days.

After trying various methods of intermittent fasting, Mosley concluded that the methods he tried were too hard physically, psychologically, and socially, so he set out to devise his own method of intermittent fasting.

The 5:2 *fast diet* that Mosley designed was based on a number of different methods of intermittent fasting.

He decided to eat normally for five out of seven days and then do a modified fast on two non-consecutive days, cutting his caloric intake on the fast days to one quarter of his usual daily calories.

Dr. Mosley chose to fast on Mondays and Thursdays because he was inspired by the prophet Mohammed who told his followers to fast not only on a monthly basis for Ramadan, but also to cut their calories for two days a week, specifically on Mondays and Thursdays.

He stuck with what he termed the 5:2 diet for about 3 months and lost about 20 pounds of fat.

His body fat decreased from 28% to 20%, his blood glucose returned to normal, his cholesterol went down, and his blood pressure improved.

His program *Eat, Fast, Live Longer* that documented his experiences of turning his health around aired in the summer of 2012. It was extremely well received and immediately began to popularize the 5:2 diet.

Chapter 3

Why Fasting is So Effective for Weight Loss and Longevity

"I love life so I want to remain young and energetic so I can enjoy it for as long as I can."

Dr. Michael Mosley

After experiencing the benefits of intermittent fasting, Dr. Mosley set an ambitious goal for himself of living longer, staying younger, and maintaining a healthy weight. The root of accomplishing this goal involved fasting. But why?

Scientists have been studying aging and longevity for decades. In the U.S., scientific research has linked food with longevity. What's particularly interesting is that scientists discovered that it's not just about what you eat, it's about when you eat as well.

During the toughest years of the depression between 1929 and 1933 food was extremely scarce. Life expectancy was projected to decrease as a result of the food shortage, but it didn't. Surprisingly, life expectancy rose by six years during this period.

Nutritionists at Cornell University during the 1930's studied the effects of fasting on animals. They discovered that significantly reducing the amount that the animals were permitted to eat enabled them to live much longer. So, could this be true for humans as well?

Why calorie restriction works

Now, more than eighty years later, science is finally starting to reveal convincing proof that there is a strong correlation between fasting and longevity. Scientists are just beginning to understand how powerful fasting can be.

Dr. Luigi Fontana, a research professor of medicine at Washington University has spent over 10 years studying a group of people referred to as **CRON**ies (**C**alorie **R**estriction with **O**ptimum **N**utrition) who severely restrict their calorie intake on a daily basis. He has discovered that these people are extremely healthy, lean, and live longer than the average person.

Dr. Luigi Fontana's goal is to understand how people can live longer without developing life-threatening diseases like cancer, heart disease, diabetes etc. He was quoted as saying "Calorie restriction without malnutrition is extremely powerful because it can slow aging and prevent many chronic diseases."

Dr. Fontana's research on organisms varying from yeast to monkeys proved that a 25-30 percent reduction in calories could increase lifespan by 50 percent and prevent disease.

According to Joseph Cordell, an avid CRONy, calorie restriction works because your body doesn't have to work as hard when you eat less. When you give your body less food it quickly recognizes that resources are low and reassigns energy from other areas towards survival, which, contrary to popular belief, is a good thing.

When starting someone on a calorie restrictive diet, Dr. Luigi Fontana begins slowly by reducing their calories by 5 to 10 percent. He makes it clear to the patient that what they eat is very important and instructs them to get the majority of their calories from vegetables, fruits, plants and nuts.

Calorie restriction enables the body to work more efficiently. It doesn't push the body to work harder than it has to. Dr. Fontana says that this is the key reason why animals on calorie restricted diets live longer.

Fasting and weight loss

It's not just about what you eat, it's about when you eat

Intermittent fasting is about timing your meals to allow for periods of fasting. It takes your body about 6-8 hours to metabolize your glycogen stores. It is only after that period of time that your body switches to burning fat. If you keep nibbling on foods during that time, glycogen keeps being replenished. This makes it harder for your body to burn fat because it is caught in a constant cycle of making and storing fat.

One of the best studies to date in support of the benefits of intermittent fasting was published in 2012 by biologist Satchidananda Panda and fellow researchers at Salk's Regulatory Biology Laboratory.

They took two groups of mice and fed each group a high-calorie, high-fat diet. The only difference between each group was when the mice were allowed to eat.

One group was allowed to graze all day and all night. The other group was only allowed to eat during an eight hour period of time at night.

The results of the study showed that both groups of mice consumed the same amount of calories but the group that had limited access to food stayed thin and healthy and didn't show any signs of chronic inflammation or high blood sugar whereas the group that had unlimited access to food gained a lot of weight and developed several health problems like high cholesterol, fatty liver disease, high blood sugar and metabolic issues.

What this means for humans is that the body can benefit from having a break from eating. Constant eating can lead to weight gain and metabolic exhaustion. Researchers suggest that even having regular meal times without grazing in between can help you avoid metabolic disease and weight gain.

Panda and his colleagues concluded their study by saying "Time-restricted feeding is a non-pharmacological strategy against obesity and associated diseases."

The most common misconception about fasting and weight loss

Ask any fitness trainer, medical doctor, or anyone that works in the healthcare industry what the optimal way to eat for weight loss is and you will likely be told to eat three small meals a day and have snacks in between. They will probably also caution you against allowing yourself to get hungry because hunger will put your body in starvation mode and make it store fat.

The idea of eating often and not letting yourself get hungry has been advocated in part by snack manufacturers, the medical community, and fad diets.

The reasoning behind this is that if you don't let yourself get hungry then you'll be less likely to overeat due to an intense desire to satisfy your hunger. The problem with this is that for many, constant snacking actually causes them to overeat.

Fasting seems rather radical and far out in a world that is sold on the idea of eating regularly to avoid hunger. The 5:2 diet considers our ancient ancestors as proof that fasting compliments the natural workings of the human body. Our ancestors didn't eat regularly rather they would hunt, kill, eat, and then have a period of scarcity before they ate again.

The reason our bodies respond well to intermittent fasting is because we evolved from and were shaped out of thousands of years of feast or famine. Our bodies work best with what they are most familiar with.

Just as the mice in the Salk laboratory experiment that were on a feast or famine regimen stayed lean, we too can maintain a lean physique with time restricted feeding.

Fasting and longevity

Dr. Michael Mosley was quoted as saying "Fasting is not about trying to live to 140 years old, it's about staying healthy for as long as you can."

Scientific research has shown a significant correlation between fasting and longevity. Most of the research has been conducted on animals, but recent studies have been done on humans as well. This is a growing field of study as scientists continue to study the effects of fasting on aging and longevity in humans.

The benefits of fasting and longevity based on scientific research

Decreased levels of IGF-1 and cell repair

IGF-1 stands for **I**nsulin-like **G**rowth **F**actor. When you have high levels of IGF-1, a protein made by the liver, then you are at a greater risk of developing many age-related diseases as well as prostate, breast, and colorectal cancer. Low levels of IGF-1 lessen these risks.

Scientists have learned by their studies on mice that a calorie restricted diet causes IGF-1 levels to drop and to remain low even after mice are put back onto a normal diet.

Professor Valter Longo is an expert on aging and studies the mechanisms that control aging. One of his studies on fasting and longevity involved two mice. One was big and had regular levels of the growth hormone IGF-1. The other mouse was small and genetically engineered to have very low levels of IGF-1. The big mouse had a life expectancy of 2 years whereas the little mouse had about a 40% longer life expectancy. In human terms that would mean that the little mouse would live 30-40 years longer than the big mouse.

Not only would the little mouse live longer, it would also live a healthier life with almost no risk of cancer or diabetes. But why is this?

IGF-1 drives cells to constantly divide. When IGF-1 levels drop, the body slows the production of new cells and focuses on repairing existing cells. Therefore, DNA damage is more likely to be repaired. That's why the mice are not prone to age-related diseases.

Longo has discovered that eating too much protein causes the cells to get locked in the "driven" mode where cells are growing too fast for damage to be efficiently repaired.

In order to slow IGF-1 levels you can eat less and consume less protein, but typically that's not enough.

Another, more effective way to lower IGF-1 is through fasting. Regular bouts of fasting can successfully lower IGF-1.

In Dr. Michael Mosley's case, a fast of 3 days and 4 nights reduced his IGF-1 levels by 50%.

Fasting allows the pancreas to rest

When the pancreas is allowed to rest, it maximizes the effectiveness of the insulin produced by the pancreas in response to high blood glucose levels. When an increased insulin sensitivity is initiated it will reduce the risk of diabetes, obesity, heart disease, and cognitive disorders.

Fasting delays the onset of Alzheimer's, dementia, and memory loss

Professor Mark Mattson at the National Institute on Aging is a leading expert on the aging brain. He conducted a study on mice that involved putting them on a feast or fast diet which Mattson called intermittent energy restriction. He found that these mice lived much longer, about the equivalent of 30 years in humans before experiencing memory issues.

When they examined the brains of the fasting mice they found that brand new brain cells had been formed which suggested that bouts of fasting triggered new neurons to grow.

According to Mattson's research, fasting stresses the brain much the same way that exercise stresses the body.

Exercise makes the body stronger by the stress it puts on it. Fasting makes the brain stronger by the stress it puts on it. This enables the brain to remain sharp longer.

These are only a few examples of how scientific research has begun to uncover the benefits of fasting and longevity. Scientific tests also show a positive correlation between fasting and chronic inflammation, asthma, stem cell regeneration, eczema and other diseases.

Intermittent fasting helps burn fat

Fat oxidation is the process by which the human body breaks down stored fat molecules (normally quite large) into smaller molecules that the body can use as energy. Without fat oxidation these large fat or lipid molecules would remain in the body adding up, unable to be used as energy.

Several hours after the nutrients of a meal have finished being absorbed by the body, the respiratory quotient drops along with insulin. When this happens the body shifts into fat burning mode. Catecholamines (hormones and neurotransmitters) flow through the blood and bind to receptors on fat cells. This activates fat mobilization which allows fat to be burned off.

Intermittent short term fasting also increases subcutaneous free fatty acid oxidation. This allows the body to burn body fat and nothing else. The optimal level of fat burning with subcutaneous free fatty acid oxidation occurs between 12 – 14 hours of fasting.

Intermittent fasting energizes the metabolism to burn fat. It also lowers the risk of obesity and improves insulin resistance.

Test studies have also shown that green tea can increase metabolism and help the body fight against excessive fat.

Intermittent fasting improves overall health and helps prevent disease

Intermittent fasting may help improve cholesterol and triglyceride levels. It may also help prevent cancer, diabetes, heart disease, high blood pressure, chronic inflammation, and stroke.

Chapter 4

How the 5:2 Diet Works

The 5:2 diet is a calorie restrictive diet that includes intermittent and modified fasting. Over the course of one week the 5:2 diet allows "feed days" and "fast days." The fast days have to be non-consecutive. How you divide your feed and fast days is up to you.

For five days you will get to eat whatever you want (the feed days) and for two days you will do a modified fast (the fast days).

Note: If you are pregnant, have compromised immunity, are underweight, a teenager or have a history of eating disorders it is important to see your doctor first before committing to the 5:2 diet. People with Type 2 diabetes should also consult a doctor first as the 5:2 diet would have to be done under medical supervision.

The fasting days

Before you start the 5:2 diet you need to decide which two non-consecutive days of the week you want to designate as fast days. These days will include modified fasting where you will cut your calorie intake to about one quarter of the calories you normally consume in a day.

Women are allowed to consume 500 calories on fast days.

Men are allowed to consume 600 calories on fast days.

Dr. Michael Mosley chose to fast on Mondays and Thursdays. He strategically chose work days in which he was less likely to think about food.

On fast days, he would typically split his allowable 600 calories between breakfast and dinner. He would normally have breakfast at 7:30am which would consist of two scrambled eggs and a piece of ham; about 300 calories. Throughout the day he would drink lots of water, black tea, and black coffee until evening. At 7:30pm he would eat a 300 calorie dinner that consisted of lots of fresh vegetables and a slice of salmon.

By doing a modified fast, Dr. Mosley allowed his body to have approximately two 12 hour periods of fasting in a 24 hour day. According to Mosley, this method of modified fasting is the most manageable and straight-forward way of fasting on fast days.

You can adjust your eating on fast days to whatever works best with your schedule, but studies have shown that a longer stretch of fasting can be more effective than breaking your 500 or 600 calories down into a couple meals and a couple small snacks in between.

Note: Fasting for prolonged periods of time (more than 14 hours) can be harmful to your health and should only be done under medical supervision. Short bursts of intermittent fasting as suggested on the 5:2 diet are ideal and actually compliment your health. Be careful not to overdo fasting. Only do what is recommended by the 5:2 diet.

The feed days

For five days on the diet you are allowed to eat whatever you want. This is where most people begin to question the effectiveness of the 5:2 diet. Why? Because it doesn't seem reasonable to be able to eat what you want and still lose weight.

Dr. Krista Varady, an associate professor of nutrition at the University of Illinois has done quite a bit of research on alternate day fasting in humans. Her method of alternate day fasting involves a fast day, then a feed day, then a fast day and another feed day. The fast days involve consuming a 500 calorie diet (600 calories for men) every other day of the week.

Through her research she has found that as long as you stick to the allowable calories on fast days you can literally eat anything you like on feed days.

One of her studies compared two groups of people on the alternate day fasting method. One group ate high-fat foods on feed days and the other group ate low-fat foods on feed days. She was expecting to see better health results in the people that ate the low-fat foods on feed days but surprisingly she saw exactly the same decreases in LDL cholesterol, triglycerides and blood pressure in both groups. This meant that in terms of the risk of cardiovascular disease, it didn't matter if you were eating high-fat or low-fat foods.

Another thing that surprised Varady about the study was that after the fast days people rarely overate on their feed days.

Defining your daily calorie count

Though you are allowed to eat whatever you want on your feed days without counting calories, you might be interested in knowing what your ideal calorie count should be on an average day.

Calorieking.com will take your age, height, gender and activity level into consideration and let you know what your daily calorie count should be.

Chapter 5

What to Eat on Fast Days

When deciding what to eat on fast days there are two key things you want to remember:

Choose foods that stay within your allotted 500 or 600 calories

Choose foods that keep you feeling full longer

Foods with a low glycemic index will help you maintain a low calorie count on fast days. Foods that contain some protein will help you feel full longer.

How does the glycemic index work?

Carbohydrates are not restricted on the 5:2 diet, but consuming the wrong kinds of carbohydrates can make your blood sugar spike and leave you feeling hungry pretty quickly.

In order to determine which carbohydrates are not ideal it's good to look at the glycemic index. Foods on the glycemic index only relate to carbohydrates. There is no relation to protein or fat.

31

On the glycemic index (GI) each food receives a score out of 100. A food item with a low score will not cause a spike in blood sugar.

There is also another kind of measurement called the glycemic load (GL). Glycemic load measures how many carbohydrates are in a serving of a particular food and how much that food will increase blood glucose. Typically you want to avoid foods that have a glycemic index over 50 or a glycemic load over 20.

Some suggestions:

Choose fish and chicken.

Limit red meat

Choose tuna, shrimp, tofu, and other plant-based proteins

Choose nuts, seeds, legumes

Choose eggs. They're always a great choice

Choose leafy greens

Choose lots of low GI vegetables

Chapter 6

Eleven Quick Tips to Help You Succeed on the 5:2 Diet

These eleven quick tips will help you maximize your weight loss and fasting efforts on the 5:2 diet. If you are diligent about following what is recommended by the 5:2 diet and sticking with your eating regimen on fast days you should start seeing results.

Note: Dr. Michael Mosley said "though the 5:2 diet has worked for me it doesn't mean that it will work for everyone. They need to do more studies on humans to prove its effectiveness."

The studies on animals and humans have shown very positive results for fasting, weight loss, and longevity but the research is still in the very early stages. Scientists will need to keep studying the effects of fasting on humans to solidly prove its effectiveness.

Tip 1

Record your current weight and BMI

Weight

Get a notebook or journal and record your 5:2 journey. First, record your starting weight. If you don't have a digital scale, get one. You need to see pounds and ounces when you weigh yourself.

During the diet, weigh yourself once a week the morning after your fast day. Don't eat anything before you weigh yourself. Keep track of your weight in your notebook. Try not to obsess about the number. You may be down a few ounces one week and then up an ounce or two the next. Don't make that a big deal. Just record the number and stick to the diet.

You may also find it handy to record what you eat on fast days. Recording what you eat and having a visual record of your adherence to the allotted calories on fast days can be a motivator. You may even want to reward yourself with a sticker or do something you enjoy that doesn't involve food in order to celebrate successful fast days.

BMI

Body **M**ass **I**ndex takes your height and weight and measures your body fat in relation to them.

The National Heart Blood and Lung Institute has a good BMI calculator online that you can use to measure your body mass index.

The BMI calculator doesn't account for age or body type so you may want to check what your ideal BMI is with your doctor or fitness trainer.

Tip 2

Get rid of the junk

Before you start the 5:2 diet, get rid of any foods that might make your fast days harder than they need to be. Yes, you can eat whatever you want for five days a week, but let's be honest, if you're trying to fast, won't it be a lot more difficult if you know there's a stash of goodies in the next room?

Some people might be fine knowing they can have goodies tomorrow after their fast day. If that's not you, get rid of the junk so it doesn't tempt you.

Tip 3

Learn how to count calories or find recipes under 500 calories for fast days

The great thing about the 5:2 diet is that you don't have to count calories every day, only two days a week on fast days if you want to.

Caloriecount.com can help you calculate your calorie intake on fast days or if you prefer, you can make things easy on yourself by having a 5:2 diet cookbook on hand that provides recipes under 500 calories. That way you won't have to count calories at all.

The recipes at the back of this book are taken from my 5:2 diet recipes book on Amazon. Calorie counts (under 500 calories) are included with each recipe. There should be enough recipes there to get you started. If you would like more recipes, pick up my 5:2 diet recipes book on Amazon.

Tip 4

Plan your fast day food

The 5:2 diet will require you to be organized when it comes to your fast days. You'll need to plan what you're going to eat on your fast day *before* your fast day. If you don't have a 5:2 fast day recipe book then you'll have to count the calories of whatever you're planning to eat ahead of time so that you stay within your calorie limit. Leaving this task until the day of your fast can easily cause you to eat more than the allowable calories simply because you'll be tempted to eat whatever's in front of you. In order to stay safe, prepare ahead of time.

Tip 5

Make a list of low calorie foods and put it on your fridge

Make a list of low calorie foods below 100, below 50, and below 25 calories. Paste the list to your refrigerator so that if you find yourself short for calories on your fast day you can refer to the list of low calorie foods and pick one that falls into your remaining daily calorie count.

Tip 6

Drink plenty of water

Make water your best friend on fast days. Drinking plenty of water and staying hydrated is important on any diet. Water can help douse your hunger by giving you the impression of being full. It can also help prevent light-headedness while you fast.

Tip 7

Make your busy days your fast days

The best way to fast is to forget that you're fasting. If you have a couple busy days in your week make those your fast days. Maybe your work schedule requires you to work longer or harder on certain days. If you make those your fast days you won't even know that you're fasting, plus the hours will pass quickly because you're busy.

As long as you can keep your mind on something other than food you'll be fine. If you don't work, organize your fast days to include a lot of activities. Make it a shopping day, cleaning day, fixing things around the house day or errand day. Anything will work as long as it keeps you busy.

Tip 8

Make your fast day dinner the goal

If you follow a fast day eating schedule like Dr. Mosley's you'll eat breakfast in the morning and then dinner about 12 hours after that. So, if dinner is your second meal of the day why not make it the goal?

The great thing about modified fasting is that you get to eat on a fast day. If it's five hours after breakfast and you're starting to get hungry don't focus on the hunger. Instead look at the positive side. You've successfully fasted for 5 hours! Begin drinking more water, tea or coffee, and focus on getting to 6 hours, then 7, then 8, with the ultimate goal being dinner! Think of how proud of yourself you'll be for accomplishing your goal. Make that feeling your motivation.

If you've ever gone for a run you'll understand this principle well. Yes, your muscles might be burning and screaming at you to stop, but you stay determined to make it to the next lamp post.

When you reach the next lamp post your aim becomes making it to the next lamp post and so on, with the ultimate goal being the completion of your run without stopping.

Tip 9

Get a 5:2 diet buddy

Being able to share your 5:2 journey with someone else can make it more enjoyable. It can also help keep you motivated and on track. Just knowing that your friend is fasting when you are can help ease the pain of going it alone. Plus, you'll be able to encourage each other to stay on track with your fast days.

Discussing your experiences, sharing recipes, or talking about fast day food ideas can also help keep both of you on track.

There's something powerful about two people with common goals working together to accomplish them.

If you can't find a 5:2 diet buddy, use your 5:2 diet journal a lot. Record as much as you can about what you eat, your weight, how you felt on your fast day etc. Writing down your experiences and feelings can help motivate you to keep going.

Tip 10

Be a mindful eater

On fast days be mindful of the food that you are eating. Enjoy the flavor and savor every bite. Be thankful for the food that you are allowed to eat that day and when you are finished eating, mindfully accept your fast as a rich opportunity to better your health. If you see fasting the right way, with a mindful spirit it won't be a burden. You can even use your fast days as an opportunity to practice mindfulness.

Fasting is an act of faith for many. Catholics fast over Lent, Jews for Yom Kippur, Greek Orthodox Christians fast for 180 days a year, Muslims fast for Ramadan, and Buddhists fast on the full moon and new moon of every lunar month. Fasting as an act of faith involves sacrifice but it is done with the right kind of spirit.

If you are interested in learning more about mindfulness I would recommend Yesenia Chavan's best-selling book *Mindfulness for Beginners* on Amazon. It will walk you through exactly how to practice mindfulness on a daily basis.

Tip 11

Enjoy your feed days

Use your feed days as a motivation through your fast days. Just because you're restricting your calories today doesn't mean you have to tomorrow.

Enjoy your feed days. Eat what you want. Love every bite of the food you get to eat. Use your feed days as a reward for making it through your fast day. Don't feel guilty for what you eat. Just enjoy it!

Chapter 7

What to Expect on the 5:2 Diet

In order to succeed on a diet it's important to know what you can expect to experience during the diet. If you know what to expect, you are more likely to stick with it when things get tough because you'll know that it's normal.

You can expect to lose one pound a week

Typically you can expect to lose one pound a week on the 5:2 diet. At first, some of this will be fat and some will be water.

You might average out to about one pound a week by losing a few ounces on some weeks and a little more than a pound on other weeks.

You can expect your body to begin to change

A few weeks into the 5:2 diet your BMI will drop and you will begin developing lean muscle mass. Your blood glucose, IGF-1 and cholesterol should all improve within a matter of weeks.

Your food preferences will change

Even though you are permitted to eat what you want for five days a week there is something that happens to people that use intermittent fasting for weight loss. Their food preferences change. They begin to lean toward vegetables and fruits instead of a piece of cake. They choose leaner cuts of meat and switch sugary high-calorie drinks for water. Healthy foods become their first choice.

Your portion size will get smaller

Intermittent fasting inadvertently trains you to recognize portion sizes that are too big. Portions that you used to eat before you started the 5:2 diet suddenly begin to look huge.

Your fast days will have taught you restrained eating. This new habit eventually becomes your norm.

Your body will take some time to adjust to fasting

If you've never fasted before it may take you some time to adjust. People who practice intermittent fasting regularly say that it gets easier the more you do it.

If you've never counted calories before, that can also be a bit of a challenge at first. But, using low calorie 5:2 diet recipes to plan your meals can relieve you of that.

You'll learn how to deal with hunger

When you experience hunger on fast days, try to remember that your body is designed to deal with a famine state. It's a good kind of stress for your body.

Hunger pangs can be aggressive and persistent but they will slowly pass. When you fast intermittently, hunger hormones known as ghrelin levels begin to normalize, reducing your feeling of hunger. This promotes human growth hormones or HGH.

HGH is the process that slows aging and plays a large part in health and fitness. It promotes muscle growth while speeding up your metabolism which causes weight loss.

At first it might be difficult to forget about your hunger but the more you fast the easier it will get.

You'll learn how not to mistake emotion for hunger

We don't always eat because we're hungry. We eat when we're bored, procrastinating, scared, needing comfort, watching a movie, or enjoying the company of others.

If you experience an urge to eat that isn't related to hunger, try going for a walk or run, taking a shower or bath, drinking tea or black coffee, reading, or engaging in any other activity that can take your mind off of your boredom, procrastinating etc.

You'll learn how to take control of your body

Fasting is all about self-control. If you're use to letting your body have anything it wants then it's going to act like a spoiled kid when you don't give it what it wants. You need to take control. Do you really want your body to boss you around or do you want to take control of your body?

With some discipline and self-control you'll be able to train your body to do what you want it to do. Be patient. It will learn your rules. Just give it some time.

You'll learn the power of having a goal

Answering the following questions *before* you start the 5:2 diet can help keep you motivated as you journey through the diet. When you know what you want and you want it bad enough you'll be willing to do whatever it takes to get it. So ask yourself...

What is your goal weight?

When do you want to hit your goal weight?

Why do you want to lose weight?

How will you feel when you achieve your goal weight?

What are you health goals?

When do you want to reach your health goals?

Why do you need to improve your health?

How will this diet help you reach your health goals?

You'll learn how to avoid triggers

Avoid social gatherings on fast days. Food will typically be served so if you prefer not to be tempted, stay away.

If you tend to stay up late and snack then consider going to bed early on your fast days.

If others in your house are not on the diet and are cooking and eating, separate yourself from them by going for a walk or run, or getting some work done in your office. That way you won't allow yourself to be tempted by the smell or sight of food.

Use common sense when it comes to avoiding triggers. Don't deliberately put yourself in a situation where you'll be tempted to break your fast.

Chapter 8

The 5:2 Diet and High Intensity Training

"I believe that we have now produced sufficient data to be able to recommend short bursts of high-intensity exercise as a safe and effective alternative to conventional workouts, removing the time barrier as an excuse for not exercising."

Dr. Michael Mosley

Exercise will maximize your 5:2 dieting efforts. When choosing what kind of exercise you can commit to during the 5:2 diet, consider what kind of exercise you enjoy and how much of a time commitment you can make.

Dr. Krista Varady tested the effectiveness of alternate day fasting and exercise on four groups of people to see if exercise would make people lose more weight while fasting. Her study revealed that combining exercise with fasting did indeed make participants drop more weight than those that just fasted.

The problem with exercise however is the amount of time that it takes. This is a giant roadblock for a lot of people because their

49

schedules don't allow them to exercise as much as they might like. If you have time to exercise a lot then by all means exercise, but if your time is limited you might want to consider HIT - High Intensity Training.

What's so special about high intensity training?

Dr. Mosley, in an effort to find a way of exercising that would fit well into his life (time-wise) and give him all the benefits of a lengthy workout discovered HIT.

He was introduced to Jamie Timmons, professor of Precision Medicine at Kings College in London who spent years researching the benefits of high intensity training.

Timmons believes that only a few minutes of high intensity training a week can improve aerobic and metabolic fitness.

Dr. Mosley wanted to test HIT himself to see how effective it was so he had some blood tests taken and then started the HIT program recommended by Timmons.

Timmons first got Mosley to pedal slowly for two minutes on an exercise bike. Mosley was then instructed to increase the resistance as high as it would go and start pedaling as fast as he could for twenty seconds after which he would slow his pedaling once more for two minutes.

After two minutes of slow pedaling he was instructed to pick up his speed once more to 100% of his ability then slow it once more for two minutes. He was to repeat this process once more for a total of one minute of high intensity training (3 x 20 seconds).

Timmons instructed Mosley to do this same exercise three times a week (for a total of about ten minutes of high intensity training a week) and repeat this for four weeks.

After four weeks, HIT had a significant positive effect on Mosley's insulin sensitivity.

Others who have done the same kind of training along with the 5:2 diet have reported significant weight loss, improved cholesterol levels, lower levels of IGF-1, and improvements in insulin fasting levels.

Mosley continued to combine HIT three times a week with his strength and flexibility workouts. His book *Fast Exercise* explains the effectiveness of HIT in detail.

Chapter 9

How to Maintain Your Ideal Weight

Dr. Mosley originally lost 20 pounds of fat on his first round of 5:2 dieting in 2012. He didn't want to continue losing weight so he switched from 5:2 dieting to 6:1 dieting in order to maintain his ideal weight.

6:1 dieting meant that he continued to cut his calories to one quarter of his daily calorie intake (600 calories) for one day a week instead of two. That way he wouldn't go on losing weight but instead would maintain his ideal weight.

He combined this with HIT and strength training and was able to maintain his ideal weight.

When you reach your ideal weight you can do what Dr. Mosley did and switch to a 6:1 diet along with exercise. This should enable you to maintain your ideal weight.

Chapter 10

30 MINUTE Fast Day BREAKFAST Recipes Under 500 Calories

Remember to stay well hydrated through the day by drinking as much water, black tea and black coffee as you want.

Tomato Zucchini Bake with Eggs and Basil

196 calories per serving

Serves 2

Ingredients

Zucchini.....2 large, chopped into chunks

Cherry tomatoes.....200 grams, halved

Garlic.....2 cloves, crushed

Olive oil.....1 tablespoon

Fresh basil.....1 small handful, chopped

Eggs.....2

Salt and pepper.....to taste

Directions

Heat the olive oil in a non-stick pan then add the zucchini. Fry for about 5 minutes until the zucchini is soft. Add the tomatoes, garlic, salt, pepper and stir. Cook for a few minutes. Make two pockets in the mixture and crack the eggs into the pockets. Cover the pan and cook until the eggs are done, about 3 minutes. Top with fresh basil and serve.

Nutrition per serving

Calories....196

Carbohydrates.....7 grams

Protein.....12 grams

Fat.....13 grams

Fibre.....3 grams

Sugar.....6 grams

Salt.....0.25 grams

Portobello Mushroom and Spinach Egg Nest

127 calories per serving

Serves 4

Ingredients

Portobello mushrooms.....4 large

Spinach leaves.....2 large handfuls

Tomatoes.....2 sliced

Eggs.....4

Garlic.....4 cloves chopped, divided

Olive oil.....2 tablespoons, divided

Salt and pepper.....to taste

Directions

Preheat the oven to 200 degrees.

Place each mushroom in an oven safe dish. Top each mushroom with two tomato slices and one chopped garlic clove. Drizzle each with half a tablespoon of olive oil and season with salt and pepper. Bake for 10 minutes.

Place a colander in the sink. Add the spinach leaves to it. Pour boiled water over the spinach to wilt the spinach leaves. Squeeze out the excess water then add the spinach to each of the four dishes.

Make a nest in the tomato garlic topping on each mushroom. Crack an egg into it. Return to oven and cook for 8 minutes. Serve.

Nutrition per serving

Calories....127

Carbohydrates.....5 grams

Protein.....9 grams

Fat.....8 grams

Fibre.....3 grams

Sugar.....5 grams

Salt.....0.4 grams

Banana Strawberry Porridge with Cinnamon

266 calories per serving

Serves 4

Ingredients

Skim milk.....450 ml

Porridge oats.....100 grams

Bananas.....3 sliced into rounds

Cinnamon.....5 teaspoons, divided

Strawberries.....400 grams, sliced

Plain fat-free natural yogurt.....150 grams

Honey....4 teaspoons, divided

Directions

In a medium saucepan combine porridge oats, skim milk, half the bananas and 1 teaspoon of cinnamon. Stir and bring to a boil. Lower heat and cook for 5 minutes stirring constantly. Divide the mixture into four bowls and top each bowl with strawberries, the remaining banana, yogurt, one teaspoon of cinnamon and one teaspoon of honey. Serve.

Nutrition per serving

Calories....266

Carbohydrates.....53 grams

Protein.....12 grams

Fat.....2 grams

Fibre.....5 grams

Sugar.....34 grams

Salt.....0.24 grams

Roasted Red Pepper, Artichoke and Basil Soufflé

275 calories per serving

Serves 4

Ingredients

Artichoke hearts.....1 – 6 ounce jar, drained and chopped

Roasted red pepper.....1 – 12 ounce jar, drained and chopped

Parmesan cheese.....4 tablespoons, divided

Fresh basil.....4 tablespoons, chopped

Eggs.....5 - separate the yolk from the whites

Whole eggs.....2

Butter.....1 tablespoon

Olive oil.....1 tablespoon

Salt and pepper

Directions

Set the oven to broil. Beat the egg yolks and two whole eggs together in a bowl. Use an electric whisk to beat the egg whites in a separate bowl.

Add the egg whites to the yolks and combine carefully. Fold in the basil, roasted red pepper, artichokes, half the cheese, salt, and pepper.

Heat the butter and oil on a pan over medium heat. Add the egg mixture and spread over the pan evenly. Cook until it is lightly brown underneath.

Sprinkle the remaining cheese over top then place the pan under broil and cook for about 2 minutes. Cut the omelet into wedges to serve.

Nutrition per serving

Calories....275

Carbohydrates.....2 grams

Protein.....19 grams

Fat.....21 grams

Fibre.....1 gram

Sugar.....1 gram

Salt.....1.01 grams

Spinach and Zucchini Ricotta Frittata

211 calories per serving

Serves 4

Ingredients

Zucchini.....2 peeled and sliced

Spinach leaves.....2 large handfuls

Ricotta cheese.....125 grams

Dried red chili flakes.....1 teaspoon

Yellow onion.....1 small, sliced

Eggs.....6

Olive oil.....1 tablespoon

Salt.....to taste

Directions

Heat the olive oil and onion on a large frying pan. When the onion is soft, add the chili flakes and zucchini and cook for 5 minutes.

Place a colander in the sink. Add the spinach leaves to it. Pour boiled water over the spinach to wilt the spinach leaves. Squeeze out the excess water and scatter the spinach onto the pan. Top with ricotta cheese.

Set the oven to broil. Beat the eggs and season with salt. Pour the eggs into the pan and cook until the eggs have partially set.

Place the egg mixture in the oven on broil and cook through. Serve.

Nutrition per serving

Calories....211

Carbohydrates.....6 grams

Protein.....15 grams

Fat.....15 grams

Fibre.....3 grams

Sugar.....5 grams

Salt.....0.5 grams

Sun-Dried Tomato and Feta Omelet

266 calories per serving

Serves 1

Ingredients

Sun-dried tomatoes.....1 – 7 ounce jar, drained and chopped

Feta cheese.....1 small handful, crumbled

Eggs.....2 whisked

Olive oil.....1 tablespoon

Salt and pepper

Directions

Heat the olive oil in a pan. Whisk the eggs in a bowl with salt and pepper then add them to the pan. Swirl the pan to coat.

When the eggs have partially set sprinkle the tomatoes and feta over half the omelet. Fold. Cook for another minute and serve.

Nutrition per serving

Calories....266

Carbohydrates.....5 grams

Protein.....18 grams

Fat.....20 grams

Fibre.....1 grams

Sugar.....4 grams

Salt.....1.8 grams

Mushroom Cheddar Omelet with Fresh Parsley and Sweet Oven Chips

391 calories per serving

Serves 1

Ingredients

Olive oil.....1 tablespoon

Button mushrooms.....1 cup, sliced

Vegetarian cheddar.....2 tablespoons, grated

Fresh parsley.....1 small handful, chopped

Sweet potato.....1 medium, cut into long strips

Eggs.....2

Salt and pepper.....to taste

Directions

Heat the oil in a pan over medium heat. Add the mushrooms and cook until soft. Remove the mushrooms from the pan and place them into a bowl.

Add the cheese and parsley to the bowl and mix.

Heat the pan once more and add the eggs. Swirl the eggs and cook them until they have partially set.

Place the mushroom mixture on half the omelet. Fold and serve with sweet oven chips.

Sweet oven chips

Place the sweet potato strips on a baking pan, drizzle with oil and season with salt and pepper. Place them in the oven at 300 degrees. Bake until soft.

Nutrition per serving

Calories....391

Carbohydrates.....0.3 grams

Protein.....22 grams

Fat.....33 grams

Fibre.....0.7 grams

Sugar.....0.2 grams

Salt.....0.9 grams

Meaty Breakfast Bake with Fresh Chives

349 calories per serving

Serves 4

Ingredients

Italian sausage.....4 - 130 gram links, chopped into rounds

Bacon.....4 strips, diced

Eggs.....6

Cherry tomatoes.....8 halved

Button mushrooms.....1 large handful, sliced

Fresh chives.....1 tablespoon, chopped

Olive oil.....2 tablespoons

Seasoning salt.....to taste

Directions

Set the oven to broil.

Heat the oil in a pan on medium heat. Add the sausage and bacon to the pan and cook until the sausages have cooked through and the bacon is crisp. Remove from pan and set aside. Add the mushrooms and cook for 3 minutes.

Put the sausage and bacon back into the pan with the mushrooms.

Crack the eggs into a bowl and season with the salt. Whisk the eggs then add them to the pan with the sausage, bacon and mushrooms. Swirl to coat the pan. Add the tomatoes and chives then place the pan in the oven to broil for 2 minutes until set.

Cut into wedges. Serve.

Nutrition per serving

Calories....349

Carbohydrates.....4 grams

Protein.....25 grams

Fat.....26 grams

Fibre.....1 gram

Sugar.....2 grams

Salt.....2.27 grams

Pistachio and Grapefruit Morning Salad

107 calories per serving

Serves 2

Ingredients

Pink grapefruit & white grapefruit.....1 of each

Pistachio nuts.....2 teaspoons, divided

Agave nectar.....2 tablespoons, divided

Directions

Divide the grapefruit segments between two bowls and top with pistachios and agave nectar.

Nutrition per serving

Calories....107

Carbohydrates.....21 grams

Protein.....2 grams

Fat.....1 gram

Fibre.....2 grams

Sugar.....12 grams

Salt.....0 grams

Chapter 11

30 MINUTE Fast Day DINNER Recipes Under 500 Calories

"The job of fasting is to supply the body with the ideal environment to accomplish its work of healing.

Joel Fuhrman, M.D.

Crab and Avocado Salad

419 calories per serving

Serves 4

Ingredients

Crabmeat.....450 grams (mix of white and brown meat)

Cherry tomatoes.....12

Avocado.....1 cut lengthwise

Crème Fraîche.....150 ml

Rocket leaf lettuce.....110 gram bag, washed

Juice of 1 lemon

Olive oil.....3 tablespoons

Salt.....to taste

Directions

Mix the crabmeat, crème fraîche, salt, and half the lemon juice together until smooth. Set aside.

Combine the lettuce, avocado and tomatoes in a large bowl. Squeeze the remaining lemon juice over the salad along with the olive oil.

Plate the salad and top with the crabmeat mixture. Serve.

Nutrition per serving

Calories.....419

Carbohydrates.....48 grams

Protein.....25 grams

Fat.....34 grams

Fibre.....3 grams

Sugar.....2 grams

Salt.....1.24 grams

Asian Salmon and Broccoli Bake

310 calories per serving

Serves 4

Ingredients

Salmon fillets.....4 fillets with skin

Broccoli.....1 head, florets only

Green onions.....1 small bunch

Low sodium soy sauce.....2 tablespoons

Juice of ½ lemon.....quarter the other half

Directions

Preheat oven to 200 degrees. Place the salmon in a roasting tin leaving space between each fillet.

Arrange the broccoli in the roasting tin alongside the salmon. Pour the lemon juice over the salmon and broccoli and add lemon quarters to the roasting tin.

Top with half the green onions and drizzle lightly with olive oil. Cook in oven for 15 minutes.

Remove from the oven and sprinkle with soy sauce then return to oven for another 4 minutes. Sprinkle with the remaining green onions. Serve.

Nutrition per serving

Calories.....310

Carbohydrates.....3 grams

Protein.....35 grams

Fat.....17 grams

Fibre.....4 grams

Sugar.....3 grams

Salt.....1.6 grams

Crème Fraîche Herb Chicken

298 calories per serving

Serves 5

Ingredients

Skinless, boneless chicken thighs.....750 grams, cut into large chunks

Crème Fraîche.....175 grams, half-fat

Apple cider vinegar.....14 ounces

Fresh parsley.....1 small handful, chopped

Fresh thyme.....1 tablespoon, leaves picked

Whole grain mustard.....2 tablespoons

Yellow onions.....2 sliced

Garlic.....3 cloves

Olive oil.....1 tablespoon

Steamed broccoli to serve

Salt and pepper

Directions

Heat the oil in a pan (that has a lid). Cook the chicken for 3 minutes on each side until brown. Remove from heat with a slotted spoon then add the onions and garlic to the pan. Cook for 3 minutes. Add the apple cider vinegar and bring to boil. Return the chicken to the pan. Cover with lid and simmer for 10 minutes.

Remove the lid and add the mustard, crème fraîche, and herbs. Bring to a mild boil and season with salt and pepper. Serve with steamed broccoli.

Nutrition per serving

Calories.....298

Carbohydrates.....8 grams

Protein.....34 grams

Fat.....12 grams

Fibre.....2 grams

Sugar.....6 grams

Salt.....0.6 grams

Sweet Steak with Barbecue Sauce

358 calories per serving

Serves 4

Ingredients

Lamb or beef steaks.....4 – 4 ounce steaks

White onion.....1 chopped

Worcestershire sauce.....3 tablespoons

Red wine vinegar.....2 tablespoons

Brown sugar.....2 tablespoon

Ketchup.....150 ml

Sunflower oil.....6 tablespoon

Salt and pepper

Directions

Heat a pan with oil on medium heat. Brush the steaks with 3 tablespoons of oil and season with salt and pepper on both sides. Place them on the pan and cook until tender.

To make the sauce, heat the remaining oil in a pan and add the onion. Cook until soft. Add all the remaining ingredients and simmer for 5 minutes.

Plate the steaks and serve with the sauce drizzled over top.

Nutrition per serving

Calories.....358

Carbohydrates.....23 grams

Protein.....38 grams

Fat.....14 grams

Fibre.....1 gram

Sugar.....21 grams

Salt.....2.13 grams

Prawn Fajitas with Creamy Avocado Sauce

320 calories per serving

Serves 2

Ingredients

Large raw prawns.....225 grams

Sour cream.....1 heaping tablespoon

Avocado.....1 roughly chopped

Red pepper.....1 seeded and sliced

Cilantro.....1 small bunch, chopped

Garlic.....6 cloves, crushed

Red chili.....1 seeded and chopped

Juice of 2 limes

Lime.....1 for wedges to serve

Whole wheat tortillas.....4

Olive oil.....1 tablespoon

A large handful of mixed salad leaves to serve

Salt.....to taste

Directions

Mix half the garlic, half the lime juice, half the chili, half the cilantro, and salt together in a bowl. Add the prawns and mix. Place the avocado, salt, remaining chili, garlic, lime juice, and sour cream together in a food processor. Stir in the remaining cilantro.

Heat the oil in a pan and cook the red pepper until soft. Add the prawn mixture and fry for 1 minute each side. Divide the prawn and red pepper mixture between four tortillas. Roll the tortillas with the mixture and serve with the salad leaves and avocado cream. Include lime wedges on side.

Nutrition per serving

Calories....320

Carbohydrates.....8 grams

Protein.....23 grams

Fat.....22 grams

Fibre.....5 grams

Sugar.....6 grams

Salt.....0.6 grams

Steak with Zesty Herb Sauce

303 calories per serving

Serves 2

Ingredients

Sirloin steaks.....2 – 125 grams each

Fresh parsley.....1 small bunch, chopped

Shallot.....1 chopped

Garlic.....2 cloves

Juice of ½ a lemon

Red wine vinegar.....2 tablespoons

Oregano.....1/2 teaspoon, dried

Chili flakes.....1/2 teaspoon

Olive oil.....6 tablespoons, divided

Salt and pepper.....to taste

Directions

Mix the oregano, garlic, chili flakes, shallot, parsley, lemon juice, red wine vinegar, and 3 tablespoons olive oil together in a food processor.

Work the remaining oil into the steaks and season with salt and pepper. Heat a pan and cook the steaks for 2 minutes per side. Remove from pan and let the steaks rest.

Top the steaks with the oregano garlic mixture. Serve.

Nutrition per serving

Calories.....303

Carbohydrates.....1 gram

Protein.....30 grams

Fat.....20 grams

Fibre.....1 gram

Sugar.....1 gram

Salt.....0.3 grams

Pork 'n Fruit Steaks

304 calories per serving

Serves 4

Ingredients

Boneless pork loin steaks.....4 steaks trimmed of fat

Chicken stock.....200 ml

Chinese five-spice powder.....2 teaspoons

Red apples.....4 cored and diced

Red currant jelly.....2 tablespoons

Red wine vinegar.....1 tablespoon

Red onion.....1 cut into wedges

Sunflower oil.....4 tablespoons, divided

Directions

Season the pork steaks with Chinese five-spice powder.

Heat 2 tablespoons of oil in a frying pan. Fry the pork for 3 minutes per side until brown. Transfer to a plate.

Heat the remaining oil along with onion wedges for about 2 minutes. Add the apples and cook for 3 minutes. Add the jelly, red wine vinegar, and chicken stock. Bring to a boil and simmer uncovered for 8 minutes until the sauce is syrupy. Place the pork into the sauce turning each piece to glaze.

Nutrition per serving

Calories....304

Carbohydrates.....25 grams

Protein.....33 grams

Fat.....9 grams

Fibre.....38 grams

Sugar.....24 grams

Salt.....0.79 grams

Pineapple Curry with Turkey Meatballs

258 calories per serving

Serves 4

Ingredients

Ground turkey.....1 pound, 454 grams

Pineapple chunks in juice.....1 – 10 ounce can drained, reserve the juice

Korma paste.....4 tablespoons (Korma paste is a mild curry paste)

Low-fat coconut milk.....400 ml can

Cilantro.....1 small bunch, chopped

Almonds.....6 tablespoons, crushed

Yellow onion.....1 chopped

Fresh ginger.....2 inches grated

Garlic.....2 cloves

Vegetable oil.....1 tablespoon

Basmati rice.....to serve

Salt and pepper

Directions

Strain the pineapples and reserve the juice. From the reserved juice keep 2 tablespoons of juice separate. Season the ground turkey with salt and pepper and shape into mini meatballs. Heat the oil in a pan and add the meatballs. Cook until brown. In a food processor blend the garlic, ginger, onion, cilantro, and the 2 tablespoons of pineapple juice. Move the meatballs to one side of the pan and add the garlic blend. Cook until soft. Add korma paste and stir together with the meatballs. Add the crushed almonds, pineapple chunks, coconut milk, pineapple juice, salt, and pepper. Simmer uncovered for 10 minutes. Serve.

Nutrition per serving

Calories.....258

Carbohydrates.....7 grams

Protein.....35 grams

Fat.....11 grams

Fibre.....2 grams

Sugar.....5 grams

Salt.....0.88 grams

Cranberry Chicken Salad

190 calories per serving

Serves 4

Ingredients

Skinless, boneless chicken breast.....2 (4 ounces each), sliced to make 4 thin breasts

Cucumber.....1/2 seeded and sliced

Dried cranberries.....25 grams

Red onion.....2 thinly sliced

Mixed salad leaves.....200 grams

Cranberry sauce.....3 ounces

Juice of 1 lime

Olive oil.....6 tablespoons, divided

Water.....2 tablespoons

Salt and pepper

Directions

Rub 3 tablespoons of olive oil on the chicken and season with salt and pepper.

Heat 3 tablespoons of oil on a pan then fry the red onion. Add the chicken and cook for about 3 minutes per side. Set aside.

Remove the chicken and slice. Keep the pan warm and add the cranberry sauce, dried cranberries, water, and lime juice to the chicken drippings and onions.

In a salad bowl, combine the mixed salad leaves, cucumber, chicken slices, and cranberry dressing. Serve immediately.

Nutrition per serving

Calories....190

Carbohydrates.....19 grams

Protein.....18 grams

Fat.....5 grams

Fibre.....2 grams

Sugar.....17 grams

Salt.....0.12 grams

Smoked Salmon with Green Beans and Chives

488 calories per serving

Serves 2

Ingredients

Smoked salmon.....250 grams

Green beans.....200 grams

New potatoes.....150 grams, halved

Olive oil.....2 tablespoons

For the dressing:

White wine vinegar.....2 tablespoons

Dijon mustard.....1 teaspoon

Fresh chives......1 handful

Vegetable oil.....2 tablespoons

Sugar.....1 teaspoon

Directions

Mix all the dressing ingredients together in a bowl.

Cook the potatoes in boiling water for 8 minutes. Add the green beans to the boiling water and cook for another 4 minutes until soft. Drain. Add the potatoes and green beans to the mustard dressing. Toss.

Heat 2 tablespoons of olive oil in a pan then add the salmon. Cook for 3 minutes per side. Plate the potatoes and beans and top with salmon.

Nutrition per serving

Calories....488

Carbohydrates.....34 grams

Protein.....24 grams

Fat.....29 grams

Fibre.....4 grams

Sugar.....3 grams

Salt.....3.83 grams

Conclusion

Congratulations on finishing the book!

Ever since I achieved my goal weight and got healthy it's been my sincere desire to share what I've learned with others.

I truly believe you can achieve your health and weight loss goals with this amazing diet. The sooner you apply what you've learned in this book, the sooner you'll start seeing great results!

All the best!

Reviews

If you received value from this book please consider posting a review on Amazon. Even a one or two line review is helpful and much appreciated!

Other Books by Gina Crawford

5:2 Diet Recipes

DASH Diet for Beginners

DASH Diet Recipes

Mediterranean Diet for Beginners

Mediterranean Diet Recipes

Sugar Detox for Beginners

Sugar Free Recipes

Paleo for Beginners

Available on Amazon

About the Author

Gina Crawford is a health and "all things natural" enthusiast and the author of several diet and health related books. After spending years of her life overweight, exhausted, and unhappy Gina made a quality decision to turn her life around. She began researching everything she could on diet, health, weight loss, and transforming her life. With dedication and perseverance she achieved her goal weight and improved her health so much that her energy level and zest for life skyrocketed. She is now on a mission to share what she learned in a concise, easy to understand, to the point kind of way that allows others to achieve maximum results in a short amount of time. Helping people live better, healthier, more passionate lives is her ultimate desire.

43594012R00054

Made in the USA
San Bernardino, CA
21 December 2016